The Half Marathon Training Program on 2 Run's a Week

The radical method for busy people to accomplish running a half marathon with just 2 runs a week!

By Mike Gingerich

ISBN: 9798606679485

Contents:

The Half Marathon Training Program on 2 Run's a Week

Is it possible to train for and run a ½ marathon when only doing 2 training runs a week?

Isn't that craziness?   Can it really work?

YES! It is possible to complete a half marathon without killing your body or spending loads of time on training runs!

YES! It is possible to be fit, prepared, and ready to run a half marathon in 12 weeks, just 90 days, doing just 2 training runs a week!

In fact, in this program you will not run over 10 miles at any time and you will be race ready to run 13.1 miles successfully and with less wear and tear on your body on race day!

What's the Secret?

The secret is 3 key ingredients:

1. Longer runs at your Half Marathon Target Heart Rate (HMTHR) during training.

2. Speedwork to toughen you up for the late miles of a ½ marathon.

3. Lots of HIIT cross-training workouts in-between runs.

Together, this combination saves you time, prepares your whole body, lessens wear and tear, and fits a busy lifestyle.

Full disclosure, I do recommend some other items as well to really help you be ready to run a ½, including a change in diet to go high protein, low carb and low sugar, cutting out processed foods and beverages, as well as stretching and feet strengthening exercises. It's a non-traditional, highly effective pathway forward for the average runner wanting to accomplish a new goal of running a ½ marathon.

What is the HMTHR?

The HMTHR is your *Half Marathon Target Heart Rate*. It's all based on science that running at your target heart rate for the race during training at percentage variations on the distance helps your body adapt and become accustomed to running at this pace.

Most training programs have you running nearly 7 days a week and heavier miles which can increase your risk of injury. As well, traditional programs use "LSD" or long-slow-distance as part of the training program which doesn't help you prepare to race, plus it is less efficient in your overall amount of time spent training!

Do I have the *time* to train for a Half Marathon?

Do you have 30 minutes most days you can squeeze in for exercise? A majority of the daily workouts can be accomplished in 30 minutes per day!

And we workout only 6 days a week. Plus, we only do one longer run per week on a consistent day, so the program can be planned around your schedule so that the "longer" day is always on the day of the week you consistently have time to do it.

Is this Program the Right Fit for Me?

This program is specifically for the recreationally competitive person who wants to finish a half marathon well, who has limited time to invest, and who wants to significantly lessen the risk of overuse injuries.

This program is **not for you** if you want to compete to win your age division, if you have recently been injured, or if you cannot run a 5k right now in under 35 minutes.

How will this work?

What I'll help you do…

Run faster, with less effort, and race your best half-marathon with much less chance of a running related injury while training the least prep miles ever! And an added bonus...You'll be an all-around stronger and more fit athlete.

Sound good? *Let's do this!*

My Story

In 2010, I was having significant ankle swelling and joint pain to the point that I could not be active and had trouble walking up stairs. I was 35 points heavier than I am now and I was not exercising.

My family doctor sent me to a Rheumatoid Doctor and I was diagnosed as having Ankylosing spondylitis or AS. I was told the path forward was simply to manage it the best they could with long term pain meds and inflammation reducing meds and that was it.

For over 2 years I did this. I was on meds daily to control swelling and I had blood work every 6 months to see how things were going. I became frustrated and discontent. Was this all there was?

During my 3rd year on the long term meds I was introduced by family to a different take on AS and the internal inflammation I was experiencing. It was a path that focused on diet changes that could reduce inflammation, and instead of refraining from activity, I needed to get active.

Within a year I was able to wean off of the AS long-term meds and I was getting active. I set a goal to run a 5K and my "training" consisted of 1-2 mile runs. I labored but finished and was hooked.

Fast forward a few years later and I typically participate in about 12 distance events a year, nearly one a month and I really don't do anything less than a 10 miler these days.   I love the ½ marathon distance and I also enjoy Sprint and Olympic Triathlons.

My journey was one of discovery, research, trial and error, refinement, and testing, first on me and later on friends and clients. Ultimately it has led me confidently to this point of writing so that I can share it with many others.

I believe there are those who wonder if they can run a ½ marathon. Those who have thought about it, maybe tried it and got injured before they got to the race day, and those who need a next step challenge...this is for you! We can get you safely and confidently to the finish line of a ½ marathon with this innovative and unique program!

I'm hooked and so are many others! Let's dive in.

The Plan:

A typical week will involve 4 High Intensity Interval Training Workouts (HIIT), a speed workout for the one run, and a "long" run (as long as we do in this shorter, efficient program) to build endurance and prep for the distance.

HIIT workouts are a combination of aerobic type exercises and strength training. The focus is on cardio conditioning, core strengthening, and muscle development. Most running programs focus on running, and leave those in them prone to injuries from overuse. Shin splints, knee aches, tendonitis and more. This program develops your WHOLE body, not just your legs and lungs, and that is the key. Less impact, work the whole body, and strengthen the entire body.

The HIIT workouts are low impact and allow for your body to recover from the runs while actively strengthening key areas in your abs, hips, and legs to help prevent overuse injuries common in the knees, ankles, and hips.   HIIT workouts require light weights based on your strength. I use two sets, a pair of 5 lb dumbbells and a pair of 10 lb dumbbells. It can be done at home, in a bedroom, or in a gym. You might want 8 lb or 15 lb, or you may start with water bottles and progress from there!

Example Workout from Week 2:

Monday: HIIT Workout - 20 minutes (Details later)
Tuesday: HIIT Workout - 30 minutes
Wednesday: Speed Workout - 3-5 miles total + Ab Workout
Thursday: HIIT Workout - 20 minutes
Friday: Rest day
Saturday: Long Run of 4 miles at HMTHR
Sunday: HIIT Workout - 30 minutes

That's the basic routine every week. Over the course of the weeks we increase distance in the speed workout up to about 5.5 miles and the long run up to a high of 10 miles in week 10.

The HIIT workouts may be tough to begin with and then over time your body will strengthen and adjust. If they become too easy, you can increase your weight used, intensity of effort, and your plank times. More on that later!

First, let's determine your Half Marathon Training Heart Rate (HMTHR)...

Half Marathon Training Heart Rate (HMTHR)

Step 1, we need to determine your HMTHR. Again, this is the target heart rate you will train at to get your body adjusted to it and comfortable with to accomplish the half marathon.

Formula:
HMTHR = Max Heart Rate (MHR) - 10k time (in minutes) + 32

Example 1. Your MHR is 170. You run a 10k in 58 minutes. Your HMTHR is 144 bpm (beats per minute). So your target heart pace for all your runs and your half marathon would be at an average of 144 bpm (range of 142-146)

To find MHR, do a 1 mile warm-up jog, then on a 400 meter track (recommended but not required) accelerate speeds every 2 minutes until you reach a maximum effort you can sustain for 2 minutes. Identify MHR at that time, you should be huffing and puffing, then do a 1 mile cool down jog. Finally use your MHR in the formula above. This will get you your "number". Your aim is to then run your workouts (other than the speed workout which uses this number but adds and subtracts for the speed and recovery) at this number.

Complete this <u>BEFORE</u> Week 1.

Your number should be broadened to a range that is is +/-5 of that number. So if you number is 150, your target heart rate range is 145-155.

Formula credit is given here to research used and shared in the *9 Mile Marathon* training program. I can recommend the book to you after you accomplish this half marathon as a next step to get you to the next level and accomplish a marathon.

HIIT (High Intensity Interval Training) Workouts

The HIIT workouts used here are from the team at HASfit. Coach Kozak and Claudia do a great job leading you through workouts and I see no reason I needed to try to recreate what they do best!

I use HASfit as my primary HIIT workout coach. While the HASfit videos are free to use on YouTube, I would encourage you to support HASfit just like you would a monthly gym membership. Reward them for the work they put in and lead you through! You can do that here: https://www.patreon.com/hasfit.

Again, the goal is to get your heartrate up and do specific routines that build lean muscle for your core and overall body. A yoga mat can be helpful and the 5, 8, 10, or 12 pound dumbells. The workouts can be downloaded and used on or offline for free. I typically do these first thing in the morning.

A 10k to Half Marathon time prediction chart is on the next page. This will help you project your half marathon finish time based on past 10K performance.

Remember, be realistic and modest in your aim. The aim here is to finish a half marathon strong, not maintain your 10k pace for 13.1 miles.

10k finish time	Predicted half marathon finish time	Required half marathon pace min/mile
1h05	2h35	11:49
1h03	2h30	11:27
1h01	2h25	11:04
59:30:00	2h20	10:41
58:00:00	2h16	10:22
56:30:00	2h12	10:04
55:00:00	2h08	9:46
53:30:00	2h04	9:27
52:00:00	2h00	9:09
51:00:00	1h58	9:00
50:00:00	1h56	8:51
48:30:00	1h52	8:32
47:30:00	1h49	8:19
46:30:00	1h46	8:05
45:30:00	1h43	7:51
44:30:00	1h41	7:42
43:30:00	1h39	7:33
42:30:00	1h37	7:24
41:45:00	1h35	7:15
41:00:00	1h33	7:05
40:00:00	1h31	6:56
39:15:00	1h29	6:47
38:30:00	1h27	6:38

Source: 9 Mile Marathon

The Half Marathon 12 Week Training Program
Weekly Plan

Week 1 (Printable Workout link at end of book)

Monday - Full Body Cross Training (at least 15 minutes & light weights of 3-12 lbs recommended) plus 2 minute Plank. My recommended workout plan:

10 minute Ultimate Cardio* - http://hasfit.com/workouts/home/cardio-aerobic/ultimate-workout/

6 minute total abs - https://www.youtube.com/watch?v=sGOMAHOJxXM or standing abs https://www.youtube.com/watch?v=bkHuvrLxpUU

2 minute Plank. https://youtu.be/py-9DiVC8tU Only take a break if you must!

Tuesday - Full Body Cross Training at least 30 minutes. Recommended workout:

30 Minute HIIT Workout - Spartan (uses dumbbells, 10 lbs typically) http://hasfit.com/workouts/home/advanced-high-intensity/spartan-hiit-workout/

2 minute Plank. https://youtu.be/py-9DiVC8tU **Only break if you must!**

Wednesday - 1 mile at HMTHR, then run 400 meters at 30+ seconds faster than race pace, followed by jogging 2 minutes at 30 seconds more than race pace to recover. 400 meters again (same speed of 30 sec faster), jog 2 minutes at 30 below; 400 meters again (same 30 sec faster), jog 2 minutes at 30 below; 1 mile at HMTHR to finish.

That's 3x 400 meter repeats in total.

6 minute total abs - https://www.youtube.com/watch?v=sGOMAHOJxXM or standing abs https://www.youtube.com/watch?v=bkHuvrLxpUU

2 minute Plank. https://youtu.be/py-9DiVC8tU
Only break if you must!

Note the Ab workout can be done at a separate time than the speed workout. I typically do the abs (6 minute and 2 minute plank) in the morning first thing and then run after or run over my noon hour.

Thursday - Full Body Cross Training (at least 15 minutes & light weights of 3-10 lbs recommended) plus 2 minute Plank.

(Recommended workout plan: same as Monday 10 minute Ultimate Cardio* and 6 minute total abs, then 2 minute Plank. No breaks. Or Substitute the 10 Minute for this 10 Minute HIIT workout with Dumbbells**)

2 minute Plank. https://youtu.be/py-9DiVC8tU

Friday - OFF - Rest your body & get enough sleep! Also, what's your diet like? You can't run well if you eat like garbage! Fresh and non-processed is best.

Saturday - Run Day! Run Day! Warm-up: 6 minute total abs, then 2 minute Plank, followed by 3.5 Mile run at HMTHR. Yes, 3.5 miles. We'll build up from this base in small increments.

6 minute total abs - https://www.youtube.com/watch?v=sGOMAHOJxXM or standing abs https://www.youtube.com/watch?v=bkHuvrLxpUU

<u>2 minute Plank</u>. https://youtu.be/py-9DiVC8tU Only break if you must!

Sunday - Full Body Cross Training (at least 15 minutes, up to 30 minutes, using light weights of 3-10 lbs recommended) plus 2 minute plank.

(Recommended workout plan: same as Monday <u>10 minute Ultimate Cardio</u>* and <u>6 minute total abs</u>, then <u>2 minute Plank</u>. No breaks. Or Substitute the 10 Minute for this <u>10 Minute HIIT workout with Dumbbells</u>**)

That's week 1. We do similar routines ahead but we build up distance and you can add more weights and then we go for tougher ab workout later in the routine. Trust the process.

Week 2

Monday - Full Body Cross Training (at least 15 minutes & light weights of 3-10 lbs recommended) plus 2 minute Plank.

Recommended workout plan: 10 minute Ultimate Cardio* and 6 minute total abs (or Standing 6 minute Abs) then 2 minute Plank. No breaks.

Tuesday - Full Body Cross Training at least 30 minutes. Recommended workout: 30 Minute HIIT Workout - Spartan (uses dumbbells 10 lbs typically). Plus 2 Minute Plank.

Wednesday - Run Day! 2 minute Plank and 6 Minute Ab workout.

1 mile at HMTHR, 3 x 400 for speed with 2 minute recover runs in-between. So, in detail: run 400 meters at 30+ seconds faster than race pace, followed by jogging 2 minutes at up to 30 seconds slower than race pace to recover. 400 meters again (same 30 sec faster), jog 2 minutes at 30 slower to recover; 400 meters again (same 30 sec faster), jog 2 minutes at 30 below; 1 mile at HMTHR to finish.

That's 3x 400 meter repeats in total with a mile warm-up and mile cooldown at HMTHR.

Thursday - Full Body Cross Training (at least 15 minutes & light weights of 3-10 lbs recommended) plus 2 minute Plank. (Recommended workout plan: same as Monday 10 minute Ultimate Cardio* and 6 minute total abs, then 2 minute Plank. No breaks. Or Substitute the 10 Minute for this 10 Minute HIIT workout with Dumbbells**)

Friday - Off - Rest that body! Trust the process. How's that diet of yours? Remember, drink lots of water daily, not a sports drink and definitely not a soda.

Saturday - Run Day! 6 minute total abs, then 2 minute Plank, followed by 4 Miles at HMTHR.

Sunday - Full Body Cross Training (at least 15 minutes & light weights of 3-10 lbs recommended) plus 2 minute Plank. Recommended workout plan:

Same as Monday <u>10 minute Ultimate Cardio</u>* and <u>6 minute total abs</u>, then <u>2 minute Plank</u>. No breaks.

Option: Substitute the 10 Minute for this <u>10 Minute HIIT workout with Dumbbells</u>**)

Week 3

Monday - Full Body Cross Training (at least 15 minutes & light weights of 3-10 lbs recommended) plus 2 minute plank.

Recommended workout plan: 10 minute Ultimate Cardio* and 6 minute total abs, then 2 minute Plank. No breaks.

Tuesday - Full Body Cross Training at least 30 minutes. Recommended workout: 30 Minute HIIT Workout - Spartan (uses dumbbells 10 lbs typically)

Wednesday - Run Day! 2 minute Plank and 6 Minute Ab workout .

1 mile at HMTHR, then run 400 meters at 30+ seconds faster than race pace, followed by jogging 2 minutes at 30 seconds more than race pace to recover. 400 meters again (same 30 sec faster), jog 2 minutes at 30 below; 400 meters (same 30 sec faster), jog 2 minutes; 400 meters again (same 30 sec faster), jog 2 minutes at 30 below; 1 mile at HMTHR to finish.

That's 4x 400 meter repeats in total with 1 mile warm-up at HMTHR and 1 mile cooldown at HMTHR.

Thursday - Full Body Cross Training (at least 15 minutes & light weights of 3-10 lbs recommended) plus 2 minute plank.

Recommended workout plan: same as Monday 10 minute Ultimate Cardio* and 6 minute total abs, then 2 minute Plank. No breaks. Or Substitute the 10 Minute for this 10 Minute HIIT workout with Dumbbells**

Friday - Off - Rest that body! How's your sleep and how's your water intake been this past week?

Saturday - Run Day! 6 minute total abs, then 2 minute Plank, followed by 5 Miles at HMTHR.

Sunday - Full Body Cross Training (at least 25 minutes & light weights of 3-10 lbs recommended) plus 2 minute plank.

Recommended workout plan: HASfit 30 Minute Full Body Workout - use 5 lb dumbbells and 10lb dumbbells, then 2 minute Plank. No breaks.

Week 4

By now you should have a feel for the routine. If anything feels too easy, add weights and intensity to the HIIT workouts. You can even test yourself with a 3 minute Plank (https://youtu.be/imbIEsULbEY) if you choose!

Monday - Full Body Cross Training (at least 25 minutes & light weights of 3-10 lbs recommended) plus 2 minute plank.

Recommended workout plan: 10 minute Ultimate Cardio* and 6 minute total abs, then 2 minute Plank. No breaks.

Tuesday - Full Body Cross Training at least 30 minutes. Recommended workout: 30 Minute HIIT Workout - Spartan (uses dumbbells 10 lbs typically)

Wednesday - Run Day! 2 minute Plank and 6 Minute Ab workout for warm-up. 1 mile at HMTHR, then run 400 meters at 30+ seconds faster than race pace, followed by jogging 2 minutes at 30 seconds more than race pace to recover. 400 meters again (same 30 sec faster), jog 2 minutes at 30 below; 400 meters (same 30 sec faster), jog 2 minutes; 400 meters again (same 30 sec faster), jog 2 minutes at 30 below; 1 mile at HMTHR to finish.

That's 4x 400 meter speed repeats in total.

Thursday - Full Body Cross Training (at least 15 minutes & light weights of 3-10 lbs recommended) plus 2 minute Plank. (Recommended workout plan: same as Monday 10 minute Ultimate Cardio* and 6 minute total abs, then 2 minute Plank. No breaks. Or Substitute the 10 Minute for this 10 Minute HIIT workout with Dumbbells**)

Friday - Off. Rest that body. Use ice if you have sore spots. Feel free to do a stretching routine. One I use for my lower back and hamstrings is here: https://youtu.be/8YXgIW9kvH4

Saturday - Run Day! 6 minute Standing Abs, then 2 minute Plank, followed by 6 Miles at HMTHR

Sunday - Full Body Cross Training (at least 15 minutes & light weights of 3-10 lbs recommended) plus 2 minute Plank. (Recommended workout plan: same as Monday 10 minute Ultimate Cardio* and 6 minute Standing Abs, then 2 minute Plank. No breaks. Or Substitute the 10 Minute for this 10 Minute HIIT workout with Dumbbells**)

Week 5

Monday - Full Body Cross Training (at least 15 minutes & light weights of 3-10 lbs recommended) plus 2 minute plank. (Recommended workout plan: 10 minute Ultimate Cardio* and 6 minute Standing Abs, then 2 minute Plank. No breaks.)

Tuesday - Full Body Cross Training at least 30 minutes. Recommended workout: 30 Minute HIIT Workout - Spartan (uses dumbbells 10 lbs typically)

Wednesday - Run Day! 2 minute Plank and 6 Minute Ab workout for warm-up. 1 mile at HMTHR, then run 400 meters at 30+ seconds faster than race pace, followed by jogging 2 minutes at 30 seconds more than race pace to recover. 400 meters again (same 30 sec faster), jog 2 minutes at 30 below; 400 meters (same 30 sec faster), jog 2 minutes; 400 meters again (same 30 sec faster), jog 2 minutes at 30 below; 1 mile at HMTHR to finish. That's 4x 400 meter repeats in total.

Thursday - Full Body Cross Training (at least 15 minutes & light weights of 3-10 lbs recommended) plus 2 minute plank. (Recommended workout plan: same as Monday 10 minute Ultimate Cardio* and 6 minute Standing Abs, then 2 minute Plank. No breaks. Or Substitute the 10 Minute for this 10 Minute HIIT workout with Dumbbells**)

Friday - off - rest body

Saturday - Run Day! 6 minute Standing Abs, then 2 minute Plank, followed by 7 Miles at HMTHR

Sunday - Full Body Cross Training (at least 25 minutes & light weights of 3-10 lbs recommended) plus 2 minute Plank. (Recommended workout plan: (Recommended workout plan: HASfit 30 Minute Full Body Workout - use 5 lb dumbbells and 10lb dumbbells, then 2 minute Plank. No breaks.)

Week 6

Monday - Full Body Cross Training (at least 15 minutes & light weights of 3-10 lbs recommended) plus 2 minute Plank. (Recommended workout plan: 10 minute Ultimate Cardio* and 6 minute Standing Abs, then 2 minute Plank. No breaks.)

Tuesday - Full Body Cross Training at least 30 minutes. Recommended workout: 30 Minute HIIT Workout - Spartan (uses dumbbells 10 lbs typically)

Wednesday - Run Day! 2 minute Plank and 6 Minute Ab workout for warm-up. 1 mile at HMTHR, then run 400 meters at 30+ seconds faster than race pace, followed by jogging 2 minutes at 30 seconds more than race pace to recover. 400 meters again (same 30 sec faster), jog 2 minutes at 30 below; 400 meters (same 30 sec faster), jog 2 minutes; 400 meters again (same 30 sec faster), jog 2 minutes at 30 below; 400 meters again (same 30 sec faster), jog 2 minutes at 30 below; 1 mile at HMTHR to finish. That's 5x 400 meter repeats in total.

Thursday - Full Body Cross Training (at least 15 minutes & light weights of 3-10 lbs recommended) plus 2 minute plank. (Recommended workout plan: same as Monday 10 minute Ultimate Cardio* and 6 minute Standing Abs, then 2 minute Plank. No breaks. Or Substitute the 10 Minute for this 10 Minute HIIT workout with Dumbbells**)

Friday - off - rest body

Saturday - Run Day! 6 minute total abs, then 2 minute Plank, followed by 7 Miles at HMTHR

Sunday - Full Body Cross Training (at least 25 minutes & light weights of 3-10 lbs recommended) plus 2+ minute plank. (Recommended workout plan: (Recommended workout plan: HASfit 30 Minute Full Body Workout - use 5 lb dumbbells and 10lb dumbbells, then 3 minute Plank. No breaks.)

Week 7

Monday - Full Body Cross Training (at least 15 minutes & light weights of 3-10 lbs recommended) plus 2 minute Plank. (Recommended workout plan: 10 minute Ultimate Cardio* and 6 minute Standing Abs, then 2 minute Plank. No breaks.)

Tuesday - Full Body Cross Training at least 30 minutes. Recommended workout: 30 Minute HIIT Workout - Spartan (uses dumbbells 10 lbs typically)

Wednesday - Run Day! 2 minute Plank and 6 Minute Ab workout for warm-up. 1 mile at HMTHR, then run 400 meters at 30+ seconds faster than race pace, followed by jogging 2 minutes at 30 seconds more than race pace to recover. 400 meters again (same 30 sec faster), jog 2 minutes at 30 below; 400 meters (same 30 sec faster), jog 2 minutes; 400 meters again (same 30 sec faster), jog 2 minutes at 30 below; 1 mile at HMTHR to finish. That's 4x 400 meter repeats in total.

Thursday - Full Body Cross Training (at least 15 minutes & light weights of 3-10 lbs recommended) plus 2 minute Plank. (Recommended workout plan: same as Monday 10 minute Ultimate Cardio* and 6 minute Standing Abs, then 2 minute Plank. No breaks. Or Substitute the 10 Minute for this 10 Minute HIIT workout with Dumbbells**)

Friday - off - rest body

Saturday - Run Day! 6 minute Standing Abs, then 2 minute Plank, followed by 8 Miles at HMTHR

Sunday - Full Body Cross Training (at least 25 minutes & light weights of 3-10 lbs recommended) plus 2 minute plank. (Recommended workout plan: (Recommended workout plan: HASfit 30 Minute Full Body Workout - use 5 lb dumbbells and 10lb dumbbells, then 2 minute Plank. No breaks.)

Week 8

Monday - Full Body Cross Training (at least 15 minutes & light weights of 3-10 lbs recommended) plus 2 minute Plank. (Recommended workout plan: 10 minute Ultimate Cardio* and 6 minute Standing Abs, then 2 minute Plank. No breaks.)

Tuesday - Full Body Cross Training at least 30 minutes. Recommended workout: 30 Minute HIIT Workout - Spartan (uses dumbbells 10 lbs typically)

Wednesday - Run Day! 2 minute Plank and 6 Minute Ab workout for warm-up. 1 mile at HMTHR, then run 400 meters at 30+ seconds faster than race pace, followed by jogging 2 minutes at 30 seconds more than race pace to recover. 400 meters again (same 30 sec faster), jog 2 minutes at 30 below; 400 meters (same 30 sec faster), jog 2 minutes; 400 meters again (same 30 sec faster), jog 2 minutes at 30 below; 1 mile at HMTHR to finish. That's 4x 400 meter repeats in total.

Thursday - Full Body Cross Training (at least 15 minutes & light weights of 3-10 lbs recommended) plus 2 minute Plank. (Recommended workout plan: same as Monday 10 minute Ultimate Cardio* and 6 minute total abs, then 2 minute Plank. No breaks. Or Substitute the 10 Minute for this 10 Minute HIIT workout with Dumbbells**)

Friday - off - rest body

Saturday - Run Day! 6 minute Standing Abs, then 2 minute Plank, followed by 9 Miles at HMTHR

Sunday - Full Body Cross Training (at least 25 minutes & light weights of 3-10 lbs recommended) plus 2 minute plank. (Recommended workout plan: (Recommended workout plan: HASfit 30 Minute Full Body Workout - use 5 lb dumbbells and 10lb dumbbells, then 2 minute Plank. No breaks.)

Week 9

Monday - Full Body Cross Training (at least 15 minutes & light weights of 3-10 lbs recommended) plus 2 minute plank. (Recommended workout plan: 10 minute Ultimate Cardio* and 6 minute Standing Abs, then 2 minute Plank. No breaks.)

Tuesday - Full Body Cross Training at least 30 minutes. Recommended workout: 30 Minute HIIT Workout - Spartan (uses dumbbells 10 lbs typically)

Wednesday - Run Day! 2 minute Plank and 6 Minute Ab workout for warm-up. 1 mile at HMTHR, then run 400 meters at 30+ seconds faster than race pace, followed by jogging 2 minutes at 30 seconds more than race pace to recover. 400 meters again (same 30 sec faster), jog 2 minutes at 30 below; 400 meters (same 30 sec faster), jog 2 minutes; 400 meters again (same 30 sec faster), jog 2 minutes at 30 below; 1 mile at HMTHR to finish. That's 4x 400 meter repeats in total.

Thursday - Full Body Cross Training (at least 15 minutes & light weights of 3-10 lbs recommended) plus 2 minute Plank. (Recommended workout plan: same as Monday 10 minute Ultimate Cardio* and 6 minute Standing Abs, then 2 minute Plank. No breaks. Or Substitute the 10 Minute for this 10 Minute HIIT workout with Dumbbells**)

Friday - off - rest body

Saturday - Run Day! 6 minute total abs, then 2 minute Plank, followed by 7 Miles at HMTHR

Sunday - Full Body Cross Training (at least 25 minutes & light weights of 3-10 lbs recommended) plus 2 minute plank. (Recommended workout plan: (Recommended workout plan: HASfit 30 Minute Full Body Workout - use 5 lb dumbbells and 10lb dumbbells, then 2 minute Plank. No breaks.)

Week 10

Monday - Full Body Cross Training (at least 15 minutes & light weights of 3-10 lbs recommended) plus 2 minute plank. (Recommended workout plan: 10 minute Ultimate Cardio* and 6 minute total abs, then 2 minute Plank. No breaks.)

Tuesday - Full Body Cross Training at least 30 minutes. Recommended workout: 30 Minute HIIT Workout - Spartan (uses dumbbells 10 lbs typically)

Wednesday - Run Day! 2 minute Plank and 6 Minute Ab workout for warm-up. 1 mile at HMTHR, then run 400 meters at 30+ seconds faster than race pace, followed by jogging 2 minutes at 30 seconds more than race pace to recover. 400 meters again (same 30 sec faster), jog 2 minutes at 30 below; 400 meters (same 30 sec faster), jog 2 minutes; 400 meters again (same 30 sec faster), jog 2 minutes at 30 below; 1 mile at HMTHR to finish. That's 4x 400 meter repeats in total.

Thursday - Full Body Cross Training (at least 15 minutes & light weights of 3-10 lbs recommended) plus 2 minute plank. (Recommended workout plan: same as Monday 10 minute Ultimate Cardio* and 6 minute Standing Abs, then 2 minute Plank. No breaks. Or Substitute the 10 Minute for this 10 Minute HIIT workout with Dumbbells**)

Friday - off - rest body

Saturday - Run Day! 6 minute Standing Abs, then 2 minute Plank, followed by 10 Miles at HMTHR

Sunday - Full Body Cross Training (at least 15 minutes & light weights of 3-10 lbs recommended) plus 2 minute plank. (Recommended workout plan: same as Monday 10 minute Ultimate Cardio* and 6 minute total abs, then 2 minute Plank. No breaks. Or Substitute the 10 Minute for this 10 Minute HIIT workout with Dumbbells**)

Week 11

Monday - Full Body Cross Training (at least 15 minutes & light weights of 3-10 lbs recommended) plus 2 minute plank. (Recommended workout plan: 10 minute Ultimate Cardio* and 6 minute Standing Abs, then 2 minute Plank. No breaks.)

Tuesday - Full Body Cross Training at least 30 minutes. Recommended workout: 30 Minute HIIT Workout - Spartan (uses dumbbells 10 lbs typically)

Wednesday - Run Day! 2 minute Plank and 6 Minute Ab workout for warm-up. 1 mile at HMTHR, then run 400 meters at 30+ seconds faster than race pace, followed by jogging 2 minutes at 30 seconds more than race pace to recover. 400 meters again (same 30 sec faster), jog 2 minutes at 30 below; 400 meters (same 30 sec faster), jog 2 minutes; 400 meters again (same 30 sec faster), 400 meters (same 30 sec faster), jog 2 minutes; 400 meters again (same 30 sec faster), jog 2 minutes at 30 below; 1 mile at HMTHR to finish. That's 5x 400 meter repeats in total.

Thursday - Full Body Cross Training (at least 15 minutes & light weights of 3-10 lbs recommended) plus 2 minute plank. (Recommended workout plan: same as Monday 10 minute Ultimate Cardio* and 6 minute Standing Abs, then 2 minute Plank. No breaks. Or Substitute the 10 Minute for this 10 Minute HIIT workout with Dumbbells**)

Friday - off - rest body

Saturday - Run Day! 6 minute Standing Abs, then 2 minute Plank, followed by 9 Miles at HMTHR

Sunday - 6 minute total abs, then 2 minute Plank. No breaks.

Week 12

Monday - Full Body Cross Training (at least 15 minutes & light weights of 3-10 lbs recommended) plus 2 minute plank. (Recommended workout plan: 10 minute Ultimate Cardio* and 6 minute Standing Abs, then 2 minute Plank. No breaks.)

Tuesday - Full Body Cross Training at least 30 minutes. Recommended workout: 30 Minute HIIT Workout - Spartan (uses dumbbells 10 lbs typically)

Wednesday - 6 minute Standing Abs, then 2 minute Plank, finish with 4 miles at HMTHR

Thursday - off- rest body

Friday - off - rest body

Saturday - RACE DAY! Half Marathon Day or rest if race is Sunday. Pace yourself. Don't start too fast. You got this!

Sunday - 6 minute Standing Abs, then 2 minute Plank. No breaks. Use foam roller and stretch.

It's a lifestyle now!

I often take a week off from running after the race to let my body heal. In the meantime, I will do the full body cross training at 80% effort to give my body some work but not strenuous training.

Take at least 2 weeks off from racing before running another half marathon. In the meantime, with this fitness base, continue your training onward starting with week 6 and align the final weeks 10-12 to sync with your next race day.

Resources

Link to Printable Online Version:

Stretching:

Lower back, Hamstring and Sciatica stretching routine: https://youtu.be/8YXgIW9kvH4

Stretch and strengthen hips with a Resistance Band:
https://www.youtube.com/watch?v=vOaq1zQ_cVc

———————————

Below are Full Body Cross Training Video _with additional Modifications by Mike._ I like to go a bit further and more intense than some of the workouts, especially once I feel comfortable with the workout. The goal is strength training and personal challenge to get better and stronger.

10 Minute Ultimate Cardio Additions - http://hasfit.com/workouts/home/cardio-aerobic/ultimate-workout/

Complete all 10 movements for one minute each at high intensity

1. Juke Move 2 x 30 sec *(Mike's add: Hold 2.5 - 5 lb dumbbell in each hand and alternate punch motion as you juke)*

2. Front Squat + Push Jerk 2 x 30 sec

3. Lateral Plank Walks 2 x 30 sec

4. Snatch from hang 2 x 30 sec

5. Reach Jumps 2 x 30 sec *(Mike's add: 2.5 - 5 lb dumbbells in each hand as you reach)*

6. Windshield Wipers 2 x 30 sec *(Mike's add: lying leg and arm raises. Use 10 lb dumbbell in each hand)*

7. Lunge + Curl 2 x 30 sec *(Mike's add: Curl on way down and on the way up, double what he shows)*

8. Bent-over Row 2 x 30 sec

9. DB Posterior Swing 2 x 30 sec

10. Forward and Back / Lateral Hops 2 x 30 sec
(Mike's add: Hold 2.5 - 5 lb dumbbell in each hand and alternate punch motion as you hop on toes)

10 Minute HIIT Workout with Dumbbells - Modifications
http://hasfit.com/workouts/home/advanced-high-intensity/10-minute-workout-hiit-workout-for-fat-loss-strength-training/
Complete 1 round of each exercise for 50 seconds each

One Arm Snatch to Reverse Lunge Catch / One Arm Snatch

Goblet Drop Squat / Drop Squat

Rotational Chop / without Weight

Dive Bomber Push Up / from Knees

Low Reverse Lunge + Squat / Reverse Lunge + Squat

Split Jack Curl / Step Back + Curl

High Plank DB Row + Bat Wing / from Knees

Upward Chop / without Weight

Crab Curl to Press

High Knee Run / Fast Feet (*Mike's Add: Use 2.5 - 5 lb dumbbells and punch as you high knee*)

10 Min HIIT Cardio Workout for Fat Loss - High Intensity Workout at Home for Women Men No Equipment
https://youtu.be/JFt0Y-6sXE0
Recommended for use while traveling (or at home to mix things up).

Full Body Cross Training at least 30 minutes. Recommended workout: 30 Minute HIIT Workout - Spartan (uses dumbbells 10 lbs typically)

See outline for routine and enhancements on the next page.

Round 1:
Lunge Push (One DB press out as lunge)
Deep Split Stance DB Row
High Plank DB Transfers

Round 2:
Warrior Lunge (DB's up and rotate)
Hammer Curl
Renegade Row

Round 3:
15 sec each side
Suitcase Squat *(add another 5lb for total of 15lb)*
Suitcase Row *(add another 5lb for total of 15lb)*
Suitcase Press

Round 4:
Iso Hip Up + Fly
Rocker to Overhead Press (Rock crunch to V-Sit, then two hand press)
Hollow Body Hold

Round 5:
15 sec each side

High Plank Reverse Fly
One Arm DB Thruster (like Arnold press)
One Arm DB Snatch

ADDITIONAL TIPS FOR SUCCESS

3 MINUTE PLANK

Are you wanting to go further and more intense with the plank portion? I have a 3 minute plan video I have done for you here (https://youtu.be/imbIEsULbEY) and as a next step beyond mine I recommend this 3 minute plank routine (plus more intense movements) from Bowflex: https://youtu.be/ynUw0YsrmSg

This is a great plank workout that steps up the intensity and keeps you on your toes.

FOAM ROLLING

For most runners, minor aches and pains are a fact of life. They accumulate over the weeks, and there's not much you can do to prevent them other than backing off whenever a minor ache pops up. While this approach is probably the best way to avoid injury altogether, some smaller ones we can roll out!

This is where foam rolling can help. Using a foam roller or tennis ball helps soften brittle muscles, so that they become more pliable, elastic, and resistant to injury.

A foam roll is like your own private deep-tissue massage therapist who never gets tired and only costs 15 or 20 bucks, one time, and lives in your closet!

WOBBLE BALANCE BOARD

One of the beliefs I have is that many of our injuries start because we have weak feet. By this I mean the muscles, ligaments, and tendons in our feet have become soft due to our over-cushioned, high back running shoes.

Because we have weak feet this causes our legs to strain and overcompensate in other areas resulting in muscle strains, hip flexor issues, sore achilles, aching knees, and more. The root is often in our feet and not the aching spot!

We need to get back to more of a natural running form, and to do that we need to strengthen our feet. Watch little children run barefoot, they have great form and no issues! I only wear racing flats to run in now to go with a low heel, low cushion approach and I do that because I continue working at strengthening my feet.

One way to strengthen your feet muscles and surrounding areas is to go barefoot more often. For those of us living in cities where this is less of an option, we can use a wobble balance board. (I got mine on Amazon for about $17 https://smile.amazon.com/gp/product/B00WJJJX2Q/ref=p px_yo_dt_b_asin_title_o06_s00?ie=UTF8&psc=1).

The wobble balance board is something I do near a wall on one leg, barefoot, daily. I stand on one leg in the middle and do calf raises on my toes, typically for a count of 30 and then switch. As opposed to a standard calf raise, the wobble board engages your entire foot (muscles, ligaments, and tendons) and you will feel it all the way up your hamstring! I do put one hand on the wall for some stability but try to focus on the one foot providing as much stability as possible.

I do this daily and it's work wonders. I've overcome achilles, knee, and hamstring issues with stronger feet!

DEALING WITH INJURY

Injuries are, unfortunately, common in runners, especially new runners. But, if you follow the guidelines and spend a lot of time foam rolling, you'll minimize your susceptibility to these injuries.

But let's be honest — you're training to run 13.1 miles for the first time. It's entirely possible that something will go wrong, and in that case, you need to know what to do when it does. It's beyond the scope of this book to diagnose injuries based on what you're feeling. The best advice I can give you is to go to a doctor, preferably one who specializes in sports medicine. I know, going to the doctor sucks, but doing it early might make the difference between being able to run your race and having to shut it down because you let your injury go untreated for too long. I go to a sports Chiropractor myself.

DON'T TRY TO RUN THROUGH PAIN!

If something starts to hurt during your training, running through the pain isn't going to do any good.

The nature of the training for a half marathon is that the mileage load will increase. So while you might be able to get through this run (or this week, or this month) on a bum knee, if you don't address the issue the mileage will eventually become too much to handle. And then you'll risk long-term damage by trying to tough it out. Don't be tough, be smart.

By the way, managing the pain with anti-inflammatories or any other drugs isn't a solution. For the most part, they'll only mask the symptoms, which will eventually lead to worsening of the injury — your body is feeling pain for a reason, and you should take it as a sign to back off a bit.

WHAT TO DO IF YOU FEEL PAIN ON A RUN

If you notice that something doesn't feel right during a run and it persists, stop when you can. If the pain is sharp, stop immediately, even if it means calling someone to pick you up.

Assuming the pain is dull and it doesn't hurt you just to walk around, take 1-3 days off and see if the pain is still there the next time you try to run. Sometimes these things have a way of working themselves out. (If it's a long run or a hard workout that's up next, you might want to think about skipping it and reworking your schedule.)

If it hurts again, it's time to do something about it.

TAKE TIME OFF

This is why I strongly believe that a training program should be flexible.

Personally, I'd start by taking a week off of running if you have an injury. Even if the injury doesn't require it, the fact that you got hurt is a sign that your body needs a break. If you simply must be active or you'll go nuts, do some cross-training that doesn't cause you any pain. But really, focus on rest above all else. During this week, see a doctor or otherwise figure out what might be going on.

In case you still haven't gone to a doctor, here's the general procedure I use to handle minor injuries.
1. Reduce training load for 4-5 days. This means adding to the number of complete rest days, where you allow your body to heal your injury, rather than having to use energy for exercise and rebuilding non-injured muscles.
2. During this time, focus on stretching (preferably dynamic), foam rolling, and icing your injury.
3. As you increase your training load again, replace some running with similar cross-training: stationary bike, elliptical machine, etc.
4. When it doesn't hurt to run anymore, resume (modified) training plan with extra stretching, foam rolling, and icing.

Pay attention to injury and back off on workouts as needed until injury is completely healed.

HEALTHY EATING RECOMMENDATIONS

DIET AND NUTRITION

This is an REALLY important area! I just do not believe you can really run well for long periods on a bad diet. Yes, I do recommend you try to "go clean" during this time period. By this I mean no junk food, processed foods (in a box, in a can, things that contain additives and preservatives), no soda pop and things with high fructose corn syrup. Those things will slow you down!

Go as natural as possible in foods. Ingredient labels should be as short as possible and you should KNOW what each ingredient is! Go high in vegetables and also moderate in fruit.

Personally, I've moved towards being Vegan. I am largely gluten free, dairy free and meat free. I am not allergic in a significant way but I notice more swelling and fatigue if I eat them, particularly dairy and processed gluten. I eat a lot of spinach salads with almonds and blueberries! I drink Soy milk, lots of water with a drop of either Peppermint or Lemon in it, and eat plenty of Almonds and organic oats. I have oatmeal for breakfast with berries or raisins. I eat plenty of rice, beans, quinoa, and tofu.

I adhere to the Eat Right 4 Your Type book to eat healthy and clean for my blood type A.

You cannot run well if you do not eat well. I'm not saying you have to be Vegan, but I am saying you have to cut out high fructose corn syrup, sugary drinks (including sports drinks), and you need to eliminate fast food and as much processed foods as possible.

Eat clean, feel better, run better! I'm serious.

Summary

That's a wrap on the 2 Runs a Week Half Marathon Training program!

It's been tried and held true for many runners. The beauty is that it enables your average person to run a half marathon, be in great shape, reduce injuries, and still have quality and balance in life.

It does not require loads of time invested. It's also flexible! You can always swap out a cross training day for another run + the abs work, or substitute in a bike ride or swim as well! It's about keeping the body moving, and doing well-rounded training versus the pounding that comes from only running. You got this!

Go do it!

I'd love to hear your results!

www.ingramcontent.com/pod-product-compliance
Lightning Source LLC
Chambersburg PA
CBHW051224250726
48655CB00006B/2583